Contents

Chapter 1 2
   Definition 2

Chapter 2 8
   What Are the Factors That Contribute to AMN? 8
   Adrenomyeloneuropathy Risk Factors 10

Chapter 3 16
   Complications that could arise 16
   Diagnosis 18
   Adrenomyeloneuropathy Treatment . 20
   Prognosis 23

Chapter 3 24
   Adrenomyeloneuropathy Prevention 24

DISCLAIMER

This information is not intended as a substitute for professional medical advice, emergency treatment or formal first-aid training.

Don't use this information to diagnose or develop treatment plan for a health problem or disease without consulting a qualified health care provider.

If you are in a life threatening or emergency medical situation, please seek medical assistance immediately

Chapter 1

Definition

AMN, or adrenomyeloneuropathy, is a disorder of the spinal cord that runs in families.

An X-linked adrenoleukodystrophy, this is a form of it. People with AMN, on average, start developing characteristics in their late twenties or early thirties. Ataxia, speech difficulties, adrenal insufficiency, sexual dysfunction, and bladder control issues are all possible signs and symptoms.

Behavioral abnormalities, vision loss, hearing problems, and/or seizures may occur in people with AMN if their brain has been affected.

AMN is caused by mutations in the ABCD1 gene and is passed down exclusively through males. For people with adrenal insufficiency, the treatment is tailored to their specific symptoms and may include steroid replacement therapy.

When it comes to Adrenomyeloneuropathy (AMN), it's clear that it runs in families.

If the responsible gene is found on the X chromosome, one of the two sex chromosomes, the condition is considered X-linked.

One of the two chromosomes found in males and females is known as the Y chromosome. Both sexes have an X chromosome and a Y chromosome, with women possessing two X chromosomes.

Because men only have one copy of the X chromosome, a single mutated copy of the disease-causing gene is all that's needed to manifest symptoms. All of a man's daughters will be affected by an X-linked condition, but none of his sons will be.

The normal copy of the gene on the other X chromosome may mask the effect of the mutant on women's X chromosome because they have two X chromosomes. Women who only have one mutation are referred to as "carriers."

Women who carry the virus typically show no signs of illness or only experience minor symptoms.

Some women, however, may be just as badly affected as men by the disease. X-linked conditions are 50% more likely to be passed down to future generations if a woman is pregnant while carrying the condition herself.

About 20% of women with one AMN ABCD1 mutation develop stiffness and weakness in their legs later in life, usually in their forties or fifties. Adrenal function is usually normal in these women.

Chapter 2

What Are the Factors That Contribute to AMN?

AMN, like ALD, is brought on by mutations in the ABCD1 gene that are passed down through families. Very long chain fatty acids (VLCFAs) are transported into cells and degraded by peroxisomes or lysosomes thanks to ABCD1 encoding the ALDP protein.

When ABCD1 is mutated, it causes a lack of ALDP, which

leads to an accumulation of VLCFAs in the blood and tissues. Myelin in the spinal cord (and brain) as well as adrenal and testes may be harmed by VLCFA buildup.

Adrenomyeloneuropathy

Risk Factors

Those who have a family history of the disease are more likely to develop adrenal leukodystrophy. As an X-linked genetic mutation, the disease primarily affects males, with some females showing symptoms but the majority being asymptomatic carriers.

Amniotic membrane necrosis symptoms

The signs and symptoms of AMN, like those of the other X-ALD subtypes, can vary widely.

Some of the symptoms that may be present are listed below, along with any necessary definitions.

- a problem with the bladder
- Peripheral neuropathy of a milder degree
- loss of weight

- Nausea
- Patients with AMN most commonly experience difficulty walking or a change in walking pattern.
- A lack of adrenal hormones such as adrenaline and cortisol, which are released by the adrenal glands located above the kidneys. Blood pressure, heart rate, and sexual development and reproduction are all influenced by these hormones. There is

insufficient production of these hormones due to adrenal insufficiency, allowing these processes to go unchecked. Seventy percent of men with AMN have adrenal insufficiency, which can be fatal.

- Impotence or sexual dysfunction may be caused by problems with the testes or the spinal cord. In the latter case, it's not all that common. Testing for the presence of testosterone in the

patient's blood can reveal the condition.
- palsy of the wrists and fingers
- alterations in behavior
- Spastic paraparesis is a condition in which the legs gradually become weaker and stiffer. This is more common in people with AMN who have the condition in their lower limbs.
- The inability to coordinate muscle movement is known as ataxia.

- Excessive muscle tone is referred to as hypertonia.
- Defects in vision
- When someone has dysarthria, it's difficult for them to articulate their thoughts or words because their speech muscles are impaired.
- Sudden convulsions/attacks/spasticity: seizure

Chapter 3

Complications that could arise

These difficulties are possible:

- dysfunction of the urinary system
- Hair loss and balding
- Anxiety attack
- a state of sedation
- Sphincter dysfunction results in issues

controlling one's bowels and one's bladder.
- Insomnia and impotence

Diagnosis

X-ALD patients with elevated levels of these molecules have AMN, which is diagnosed with a simple blood test that measures the amount of very long chain fatty acids in the blood. There is also a blood test based on DNA.

If an X-ALD blood test comes back positive, a magnetic resonance imaging (MRI) scan will be ordered to see if there is any cerebral involvement. Adrenal insufficiency is also a common symptom of the disease that can be treated, so the patient will undergo another blood test to check for it.

Adrenomyeloneuropathy Treatment

There is no cure for AMN at this time, but patients can find relief from the disease's symptoms through clinical and dietary treatments.

Adrenal insufficiency is a symptom that can appear in patients with AMN. In the upper part of the back, just above the kidneys, you'll find the adrenal glands, which produce adrenaline and cortisol. Blood pressure, heart rate, and sexual development and reproduction are all influenced by these hormones. There is insufficient production of these hormones due to adrenal insufficiency, allowing these processes to go unchecked. Steroid replacement therapy can correct adrenal insufficiency and generally improve the patient's quality of life. Adrenal insufficiency can be fatal if it is not detected and treated in time. There is no need for "pharmacologic" doses of steroids; only replacement dosages, which

have none of the side effects,
are needed.

Prognosis

For those suffering from adrenomyeloneuropathy (AMN), the prognosis varies depending on the specific subtype.

There is a worse prognosis for AMN patients who have cerebral involvement. Physical therapy, bladder control management, and counseling can all help people with and without cerebral involvement live fulfilling personal and professional lives.

Chapter 3

Adrenomyeloneuropathy

Prevention

If one or both parents have a history of X-linked adrenoleukodystrophy, couples should seek genetic counseling. A mother's chance of carrying the disease is 85% if her son has it.

There is also a prenatal test for X-linked adrenoleukodystrophy. Cells from the chorionic villus or amniocentesis are tested. These tests look for a known genetic change in the family or very high levels of long-chain fatty acids.

Other Books by Author

1. getbook.at/SCHIZOPHRENIA
2. getbook.at/FLACCID-ACUTE-MYELITIS
3. getbook.at/THE-LUPUS-GUIDE
4. mybook.to/BRAIN-ANEURYSM
5. mybook.to/AMYOTROPHIC-SCLEROSIS
6. mybook.to/CHILDRENSCHIZOPHRENIA

www.ingramcontent.com/pod-product-compliance
Lightning Source LLC
Chambersburg PA
CBHW030041230526
45472CB00002B/619